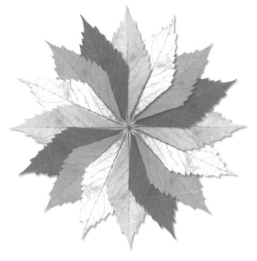

autumn winter spring summer

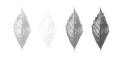

autumn winter spring summer

sandra sabatini

silvia mori

chloë fremantle illustrator

monica smith foreword

ann colcord translator

pinter & martin

Pinter & Martin

autumn, winter, spring, summer
yoga through the seasons

First published in Italian as Lo yoga nelle stagioni
in 2004 by Edizioni L'Età dell' Acquario

This revised English language edition first published by Pinter & Martin Ltd 2008

A catalogue record for this book
is available from the British Library

ISBN 978-1-905177-10-3

Printed in Great Britain by
TJ International Ltd, Padstow, Cornwall

Pinter & Martin Ltd
6 Effra Parade
London SW2 1PS
www.pinterandmartin.com

To *Lorenzo, Chiara, Michele
Simone* and *Margherita*
our children

acknowledgements

We would like to express our gratitude and recognition of the great stream of the Indian and Chinese texts and masters which have nourished us and continue to provide a daily source of understanding.

To Thich Nhat Hanh for teaching us the peace in every footstep.

To Vanda for showing us the way.

To all the students and travelling companions who have helped us grow with their trust and support.

A special thanks to Ann, Monica, Martin & Maria. And a special thank you to Chloe for her illustrations that express so beautifully the flow of movement in the practice of yoga. Without her contribution this book would not exist.

contents

preface: re-enchantment

Poetry draws us into a land of enchantment. Everything looks sparkling and new, like sunshine following the rain. Poetic words give us a sense of the creative source of our experiences and bring new energy.

Sandra and Silvia's experiments restore enchantment to yoga, and offer a way to bring daily practice into an 'enchanted space'.

Sanskrit is the mother tongue of yoga, a poetic language that was once sung. Then as now, the words for the practice of yoga are evocative and musical.

We can think of the inner dimension as a fountain or spring which can relieve thirst. In yoga we draw from that source where it is flowing, where the archetypes of the asanas come to life, where vitality releases the bud into flowering, animates the body and awakens the spirit.

This book is a dialogue at the source of yoga, where it flows into attentive matter and brings it to life, and breathes it into motion.

The vital energy that courses through the seasons, shaping the landscape and influencing the body also shapes us from within.

Yoga attuned to the seasons offers a way to heed the body, not to force it, but to lovingly attend to its intimate nature. Yoga nourishes through simplicity, through small imperceptible movements the seasons suggest, restoring us to health … We observe changes in nature, seeds sprouting, water dripping on an autumn leaf. We allow ourselves to be sustained by the embrace of the earth, taste, savour, sniff, touch, perhaps sleep … in a ray of sunshine.

We are encouraged to move very gently, one level at a time, shedding our skins, breathing, imitating the buzzing of bumble bees sitting under the branches of a flowering apple tree. Slowly we discover how to see as if for the first time, how to open ourselves to sense … with our whole body.

I read the text as if I were rereading my diary, to find myself again.
I recognise the flow of thoughts under the surface of daily concerns and steady demands on my time and energy.

I feel linked with a river which flows deep and close to home and which brings us all together and connects us somehow on a subtle level.

The rhythm of language, like a pulse, releases images, sensations, personal suggestions which are also universal, and on this level simply records the path of the body in the course of the year.

A mind busy with plans and projects for getting things done creates a great deal of static, feels pressed for time, fills all the spaces. Silence is banished, and there is no sense of listening within to what is happening below the surface. My path. It needs some external method to reach me, like this book. The text gracefully suggests images, movements, ways of breathing … we can entrust ourselves to its guidance season after season.

It is so rare to hear anything about our needs. We tend to make demands on our bodies, but it is also imperative to consider our other needs. But nature works in a completely different way and we are part of nature.

'An ounce of prevention is worth a pound of cure', and getting in tune with the nature within and surrounding us goes through stages of awareness, signs or symptoms, dreams, fragrances, creaks and squeaks, the shifting of underground currents.

Finding a place for observing what is happening, verifying day after day the silent presence of the ground and its unceasing sustenance and support, we encounter a sense of trust and trust brings the assurance of being able to do what is needed.

The wings and the air, the land and the water, the leaves and the sun, the bee and the flower, everything is the way we thought of it in childhood – a dance. Reading this book, season after season, and practicing as the days go by, will enchant.

Monica Smith

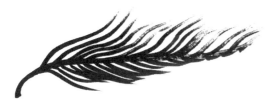

around the seasons with yoga

This is a four-handed book ... a joint experiment ... two voices recounting experiences and reflections connected with practicing and teaching yoga. Focusing on the seasons rekindles our relationship with nature, which may slip out of awareness. Writing about the seasons prompted us to consider practice as a search for harmony, encouragement, a key for getting closer to the roundness of the seasons.

During a retreat with Thich Nhat Hanh we discovered the beauty and simplicity of walking meditation. We became more aware of yoga as a practice that enables us to find the sense of rhythm and a deep connection with earth, air, sunlight ... a dialogue between the body and its surroundings, opening our awareness to changing beauties and their flow.

The seasons nudge us to dust off habits, introduce new insights which can enrich our practice.

This book starts with autumn and goes through the four seasons. The earth appears and disappears: it is at the centre of everything, everything moves around it, it is actively present. We can expand only after we have sensed our contact with the ground and its constant support. It is the source of our roots.

Our practice found inspiration and support in the huge stream of the Chinese tradition: we learned how much interconnected we are with the cycles of the year, the small and the large cycles. In every season energy tends to have its own special quality and move in a particular way: the gathering together and withdrawal of energy from the surface in the autumn, the silent stillness of winter, the push to emerge and grow in the spring, the expansive exuberance of summer.

Each season according to that tradition is divided in three phases: one that leads you toward the incoming season, one that represents the core of it and one that takes you by the hand and guides you out of it. This is why we propose three short sequences of asana and breathing patterns for each season. Acceptance of their dance will refine our perception and bring us clues on how to follow them.

'Health doesn't make a sound' but needs a range of different forms of attention like standing, walking, breathing, relaxation and meditation, which help us to tune our inner sound with the sound of the universe. These sharpen our capacity to hear and to listen, and bring balance.

Yoga positions in the open air, amidst stones, grass, ants, pine needles, puffs of wind, light flickering on some leaves, brings vividness to our practice and arouses our senses. Letting the eyes settle on an expanse of sea, and its natural motion, or the way the sunlight touches a petal or a leaf can strike deep inner chords.

The chapter **footsteps** offers a key to move through the sequences later proposed, the focus on our roots, our connection with the Earth and how to move towards it. Observing our standing position as if it were a totally new experience may disclose interesting surprises and new insights. And during the yoga practice, the coming back over and over again to this still observation may invite a calm and easy flow of breath that takes us into a state of quietness and lightness.

We would like this book to offer a series of simple positions with different breathing rhythms for experiment and play. The various parts of this dance stir something that may be dormant or dozing. Energy can start moving again and bring new balance and understanding.

Sandra Sabatini & Silvia Mori
Campiglia, July 2007

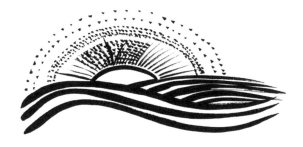

'Nature' is what We see –
The Hill – the Afternoon –
Squirrel – Eclipse – the Bumble bee –
Nay – Nature is Heaven –

'Nature' is what We hear –
The Bobolink – the Sea –
Thunder – the Cricket –
Nay – Nature is Harmony –

'Nature' is what We know –
But have no Art to say –
So impotent our Wisdom is
To Her Simplicity.

EMILY DICKINSON

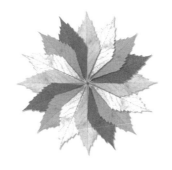

autumn winter spring summer

footsteps

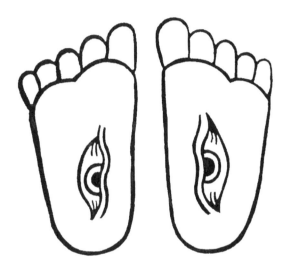

The practice of yoga encourages a dialogue
between our feet and the earth
Without this reciprocal dialogue the practice
loses direction and becomes superficial.
So we approach every season
through listening to our footsteps.

This very simple and ancient activity creates
an immediate resonance within us.
It is with the feet that we travel through
the seasons and the places of the world,
and it is through the feet that we
may start to refine our perceptions.

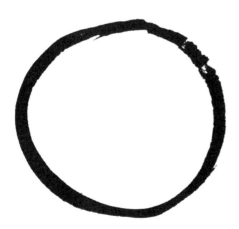

on waking up

still in bed invite your feet to spread out gently
from the centre as if they were yawning
let the yawn travel all the way down the spine
to the soles of the feet …
repeat several times so that the journey acquires clarity and ease …
the journey that takes you from deep sleep
to the threshold of awakening is a long one

let it be gradual

then, let the breath flow all the way down to one foot
like a river streaming down to the valley a few times …
and encourage a similar flow to the other foot …
feel how differently they respond to the touch of the breath …

wait …

now let the message roll towards the soles of both feet
at the same time
feel that the gentle touch spreads and awakens
the intelligence of both feet
as your perception becomes more vivid,
slowly extend the heels and then spread out the toes
without any effort

relax and welcome the new day with a new in-breath

footprints

lazy afternoon
a fly explores
the shape of my feet

as you stand, accept the request from the ground
to let the feet drop and entrust them to the Earth below
welcome the embrace that comes from the ground as
it reaches your feet and encourages your heels to sink
feel how you are standing on your own two feet
nowhere to go
nothing to do
see if you can drop the weight through the hips
down into the feet and on into the ground

see if you can accept the invitation to become taller
that seems to follow
continue to explore the vast range of possibilities
as you continue to stand and relax
as you drop the weight let any unnecessary tensions go as well

the invitation that comes from the Earth is very seductive
it brings a sort of subtle oscillation into the standing pose
let your body go through all the minute adjustments
without stiffening the ankles, knees or feet

the pull of gravity offers a stream of awareness that spreads from
the centre of the feet to the heels and to the toes, widening each sole
no hurry, no rush
wait
allow time to renew the connection to the Earth through your feet
over and over again
the feet become playful and sensitive to the contact with the Mother Earth

let your body float through all the changes brought about
by the widening of the base
enjoy the subtle dance of adjustments that brings
a special sense of ease
let your body sway
as you surrender to the tiny adjustments introduced by breath and gravity
the body starts to feel grateful that the feet are so firmly planted
on the ground and glad to discover the sense of lightness
that expands through the upper part of the body

if your body is inquisitive enough to play with balance,
you will soon experience a natural inner alignment
between Heaven and Earth

gather energy from the earth

dewy grass
bare feet
tingling with memories

find a quiet spot, either inside or outdoors, where it's possible to
remove not only your shoes but also your socks, and place both feet
in alignment, not close together but not too far from each other
check that the toes point straight ahead and not to the side
relax the body
then scan the body, starting with the head, moving your attention
down and inside the joints, releasing and allowing space, along the
arms to the tips of the fingers and down the legs to the tips of the toes

relax your gaze, keep the eyes open and look around
without focusing on any detail …
let the eyebrows lengthen out to the sides …
release the facial muscles and especially the jaw …
the mouth is soft …
the lips touch gently …
the nostrils release to let the air pass through effortlessly …

just listen to the contact of the soles of the feet on the ground
for a few moments

how does the right foot feel on the ground …
what is the shape of the foot …
how does the weight land, and where …
how strong is the outer edge of the foot …
what is the impact of the foot on the ground …
how free are the toes to elongate …
can the inner part of the foot spread to activate that point
called 'the Sparkling Spring'
that is the point of contact with the Energy of Mother Earth
under and around me …
then bring the same amount of time and attention to the left foot…
extend your perception to both feet together,
breathe in, breathe out calmly …
feel your roots connecting with the Earth …
deep roots … full of vitality

on slow walking

slow down your pace until each step
becomes the focus of your practice
let the back foot slowly leave the surface of the Earth
slowly as if the roots underneath are still pulling ...
first the heel, then the centre of the sole, then the base of the toes
let the foot travel through space until it lands on the Earth again
and sinks down into it

the sole widens ...
the outside of the foot eagerly spreads ...
the toes fan open ...
from the base of the little toe the movement ripples
to the base of the big toe
the inner arch springs to life and now the back foot gets ready
to leave the stability of the Earth and venture through space
and then ...
with great relief ...
connects with the Earth again

at first each tiny step seems to undermine
the steadiness of the standing position
its subversive motion shakes your being
relax … let go … accept it …
the next step brings you into the future
and the previous one is already past …

let your gaze rest in the far distance while
the attention is vividly present in each and every step
walking becomes more rhythmical …
the loss and regaining of balance less abrupt …
each step continues to require your full attention
a joyful presence that never turns into tension …
no stiffness, no holding …

small steps where the feet touch the ground
with respect and loving care
as the walking becomes pleasantly easy
you can feel the inhalation springing up from one foot
and the exhalation streaming down and out
through the opposite foot

to inhale is to absorb the strength of the Earth
and to exhale is to reconnect with it over and over again

walk slowly in silence,
delighted by the rhythm of the breath
and the peacefulness inside and around you

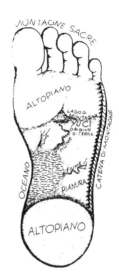

hands on feet

touching the feet –
gentle massage brings
increased awareness and vitality

a gentle foot massage is a good way to start your practice, especially in
the evening, after a busy day, when the head is already full of strands of
thoughts and images, and quietness is welcomed
first rub the palms of the hands together, many times, until they are
warm and vibrant and ready to share their radiance with the feet
stroking both sides of the foot gently, feel you are able to touch not only
the skin but deep inside the wonderful structure of the foot, with its
innumerable tiny muscles and ligaments and small strong bones
explore the quality of the two arches of each foot: the inner arch,
that big arch with curves reconnecting to those of the spine,
and the outer arch, that bony ridge that in some ancient Chinese maps
is called 'the chain of mountains'
surely those map makers were stressing the importance of the arches
for the balance of the whole body, its strength and its need for roots
down into the earth

then pinch the Achilles tendon with thumb and index finger repeatedly,
and then follow it up from the ankle until it disappears into the calf
muscle, pinching it as you go to make it more and more powerful ...

resting the fingertips on the base of the toes, rub the heel and the sole of
the foot, sense its vitality, its sensitivity, and slowly open the tissues around
the central spot behind the toes[1], 'the sparkling spring' that gathers energy
from the planet and enables us to discharge toxins from our bodies

on that very spot, press with the thumb, following the rhythm
of the breath, inhale and rest, exhale and press gently but firmly
continue doing this until the spot feels alive,
responding to the touch of your thumb
be attentive to the skin between the toes
smoothly pinch the flesh there and rub it with your fingers, as if removing
dust and grime
the traditional name for this part of the massage is
'pulling away the mud'
it helps to remove toxins which lodge there and to return them to the
blood/lymph circulation system so that the body can eliminate them

deep energy vessels radiate inside those tiny spaces between the toes,
and this is a way to encourage the flow of Qi [2]
so pull away the mud from the toes mindfully and carefully …
and then elongate each toe one at a time, pinching the tip,
allowing space in the joints …

after massaging both feet hold your arms out in front of the body and
lightly shake both hands as if you are shaking water from them
and sending it to the horizon …

then pause for a while, sitting cross legged,
and become aware of how your feet feel now …
their connection with the whole body …

that path is you
that is why it will never tire of waiting
whether it is covered with red dust,
autumn leaves,
or icy snow,
come back to the path.
you will be like the tree of life
your leaves, trunk, branches,
and the blossoms of your soul
will be fresh and beautiful,
once you enter the practice of Earth Touching

THICH NHAT HANH

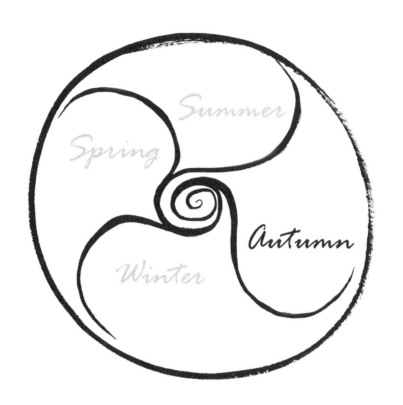

white dew

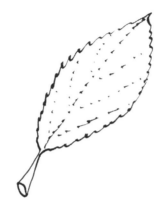

outside

walk and listen to the sound of the footsteps
walking on the grass
walking on fallen leaves
the sound of footsteps on gravel …
on pavement …

breathe while listening …
without any sense of hurry
sense the feet walking …

listen to the sound of the breath and the footsteps

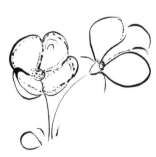

standing

with the feet parallel under the hips
let them settle down

keeping the contact with the ground
exhale ... inhale ...
letting the roots grow down into the ground
deep and thick ...
and the head blossom above the body
like a flower on a stalk ...

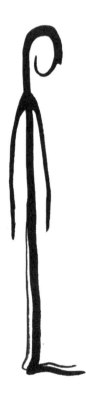

exhale and let the body lengthen forwards ...
sense the way the upper back releases ...
all the back of the body,
from the neck to the heels ...
the knees stay soft, the feet open
and come up with an exhalation
letting the spine straighten bit by bit
with the head last

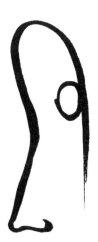

repeat this several times ...
letting the upper back unroll as it bends forward ...
breathe ...
letting the heels sink into the ground
return to upright with an exhalation

standing

with more distance between the feet
breathe and let roots grow into the ground as you exhale

breathe in and let the spine find its length ...
breathe out and lengthen forwards ...
let the breath flow in and out
and with an exhalation return to standing
with the head poised on top

repeat several times

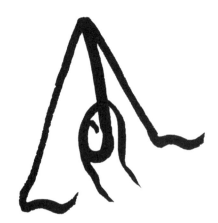

face down on the ground

with the front of the body in contact with the ground
slowly let the arms extend beyond the head

breathe and let go
take time to sense the letting go
breathe
feel the spine soften and release ...

how good it feels to let go, to release tension,
and let stiffness and tightness slip away ...

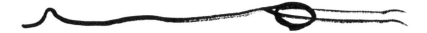

slowly bring the arms to rest by the sides of the body
listen to the flow of breath ...
the legs become heavy, the big toes touch

then put the hands under the forehead
so the neck can find its length ...
the breath goes more deeply into the body ...

sitting on the heels

place one hand on the abdomen
and the other on the sacrum ...
the warmth of the hands draws
breath into the pelvis ...

then lengthen forwards
with the forehead towards the ground
and listen

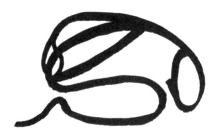

return to a vertical position
sitting with the spine long
and interlace the fingers with both hands on the sacrum

let the forehead move towards the ground again
let the arms rise up behind
getting longer and higher
release the arms
and rest the palms of the hands on
the ground letting weariness and
tension flow out and away …

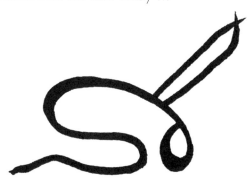

breathing with short pauses

lying on the back
with knees bent,
the feet wide and in full contact with the ground …
inhale gently
and while exhaling pause briefly
and focus attention on the upper back
between the shoulder blades …
continue the exhalation
down to the rim of the pelvis,
the space at the back of the waist
and linger there …
complete the exhalation
pausing briefly at the sacrum …
inhale delicately …

spend a few minutes exploring
this ancient breathing practice
which awakens fuller awareness in the spine

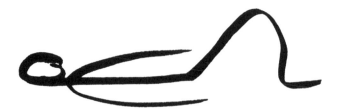

brief relaxation on the ground

feel the heaviness of the head as it gives in to the ground

the shoulders sink gently down,
the arms flop
the pelvis becomes heavy
the legs shed their weight into the ground

let go completely
and feel the support of the earth

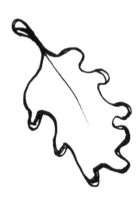

in the midst of autumn

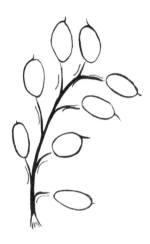

swinging

standing, let the arms begin to swing,
with more space between the feet
knees loosely bent
arms hanging limp
let them start to swing around the body
the rhythm comes from the ground,
the knees respond with a gentle springiness ...
the arms swirl around the body
the movement takes over ...
the eyes follow the swinging,
towards the right and towards the left
and towards the back,
watching to see what passes before the eyes,
the glance softly focused ...

the movement eventually comes to an end ...
return to the centre,
resting the hands above the navel
and listen to the breath...
feel the force of gravity,
present in the feet,
the legs, the pelvis ...

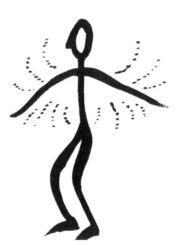

standing

bring attention to the upper back
and its connection with the ground again
through the heels
while the top of the head
connects with the sky ...

letting the movement come from the spine
let the arms and hands extend out at the sides ...
inhale and open the palms of the hands ...
exhale and turn them,
so that the palms of the hands face backwards ...

let the movement follow the flow of the breath
and harmonise with the rhythm of
exhaling and inhaling

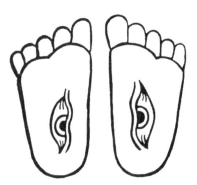

standing

with the hands together behind the back
and the fingers interweaving
lengthen forwards and down ...
slowly letting the body go
and the head drop

and let the arms lift ...
while the soles of the feet
sink into the ground ...
without any hurry, exhaling,
bend the knees slightly, and come up

a few breaths
then exhaling bend forward again,
lengthening,
inhale sensing the spine
exhaling return to standing ...

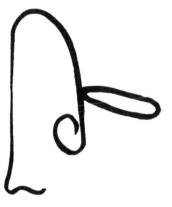

on your front

join the palms of the hands in front of the heart …
inhaling, let them lift towards the sky …
exhaling, let them return down in front of the heart …

exhaling, bring the forehead towards the ground
let the spine lengthen
without any hurry …

slide the whole body down to the ground
let the breath flow smoothly
and let the body contact the ground
from the fingertips to the toes …
breathing

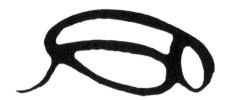

lying face down on the ground

bring the arms along the outside of the legs

with the palms turned up …
the jaw relaxed, the neck releasing …
follow the movement which comes spontaneously
with the exhalation …
rising up …

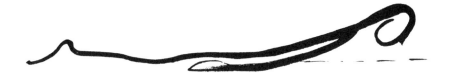

shift the position of the hands to the sides of the chest
let them give support, releasing the fingers
the elbows move closer to each other …
listening to the breath

wait for the in-breath and the out-breath
to encourage a wave-like movement
along the upper back …
receive this wave and sense how the back responds
to this wave and is transformed by the flow …

return to the ground
without losing the quality of attention to the breath,
to the movement along the spine …
slowly …

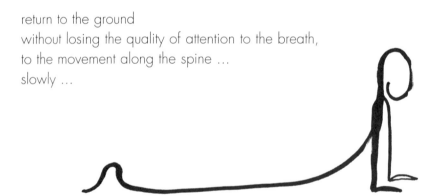

repeat several times

standing

with the feet parallel under the hips
sensing the contact with the ground
lengthen forwards keeping the legs soft,
weight flowing through the legs
into the feet and into the ground ...

the hands may touch the ground and rest there ...
the spine releases
    and lets any stiffness and tension go
      the neck becomes soft
       and the head drops any weariness or sense of effort

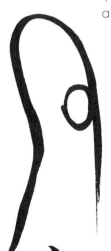

      continue to trust the feet entirely
      without letting weight go into the hands ...

      exhaling, let the outside of the ankles lengthen down ...
      inhaling, feel the arches on the inside
      of the feet reawaken

sitting with crossed legs

in the easiest way,
with one foot in front of the other ...
gently inhale ...   gently exhale ...

make a brief pause
and focus the attention between the shoulder blades ...
relax the shoulders ... continue exhaling
and when the breath reaches the rim of the pelvis
pause briefly ...

let the weight of the pelvis sink into the ground
complete the exhalation ...
focus attention on the sacrum with another small pause ...

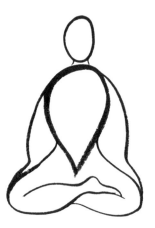

inhale delicately
repeat for several minutes
getting into the rhythm ...
where the pauses offer rest and suspension
no trace of effort ...
exhale

the inhalation begins at the sacrum and rises towards the waist
with a brief pause let the pelvis release ...
follow the path of the inhalation up between the shoulder blades
with a brief pause let the shoulders release ...
finish the inhalation towards the top of the head ...
slowly become empty with an exhalation ...

repeat for several minutes ...

then lie on the back

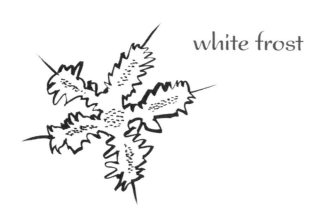

white frost

standing

shift the weight from the centre of the feet
towards the base of the toes ...
from there towards the heels ...
let the heels sink more deeply into the ground
and free the toes ...
exhale ...
the centre of the foot opens ...
inhale ...

the energy from the ground rises
through the centre of the feet up to the crown
of the head ...
play with these sensations until
the breath and the movement harmonise ...

take a step forward
the arms rise up, over the head ...
lightly ...
moving from the upper back, like wings ...
with the breath ...
when they feel tired they rest
and drop down next to the thighs

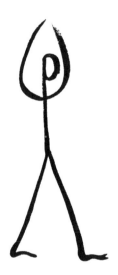

find stability and balance …
exhale and imagine the feet growing roots
deep into the ground …

the front knee slightly bends …
inhaling, the arms rise up towards the sky …
the palms of the hands join …
then the hands move down in front of the heart
pause and listen to the breath …

let the arms go up again
in lightness …
in space …
while the feet stay large
and stable …

repeat the sequence
on the other side without hurry …
it will be different …

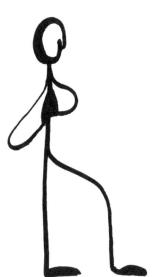

with an exhalation
lengthen forwards …
the toes continue
to be free of weight …
the back of the knees
is open but not tight …
the neck is in continual dialogue
with the sacrum …
as if offering something precious
the elbows move closer together
the arms extend forwards
the palms of the hands face the sky …

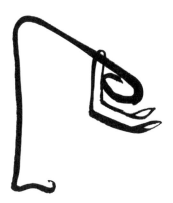

with an exhalation lengthen the heels simultaneously
towards the ground,
slightly bend the knees
and return to standing …
feeling drawn by the earth

on the ground

the arms are long in front of the head …
the front of the body rests on the ground …
breathing …
filling the body with calmness …
exhaling tiredness into the ground
inhaling lightness …
the spine has no weight …
it ripples …

eventually the upper part of the spine rises up from the ground …
the arms follow …
the elbows slide down and rest on the ground …
the breath follows the movement
along the entire spine

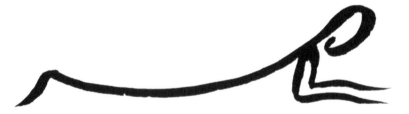

alternate nostril breathing

sitting with crossed legs
touch the soles of the feet …
change the position of the legs several times …
encourage the feet to turn
so the soles start to face up …
with the right ring finger close the left nostril
and inhale through the right …
with the thumb close the right nostril
and exhale through the left

close on the left and inhale on the right and vice verse
continue to alternate effortlessly …
letting the sound and the rhythm of the breath become calm …
silent …

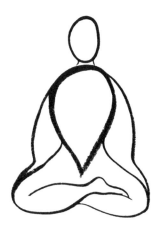

allowing several minutes to get into this rhythmic breathing ...
alternating brings vitality ...
before changing the position of the legs
turn and look to the right
inhale and raise the right arm ...
exhale and reach behind
the spine for the right foot ...
wait for the base of the body to become heavy
and the spine light and free ...

changing the position of the feet
repeat on the other side ...
continue the breathing
until the back becomes lighter ...

then lying on the back for the relaxation
which completes the practice ...
an important time ...
attention is still on the breath,
on the subtle movement within that has been sensed

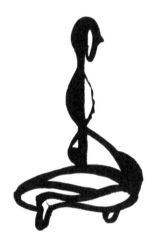

relaxation in the autumn

lying on the back,
feel all the points where the body touches the ground ...
sense the contact the neck finds with the ground ...
and the places where the right arm contacts the ground ...
and the left arm ...
the right leg ...
the left leg ...

with an exhalation let the heels go ...
let your attention trace the back of the whole body several times ...
from the top of the head to the heels ...

with full awareness pause to touch all the places
where the body rests on the ground ...

as the relaxation deepens let this dialogue
between the body and the ground continue ...

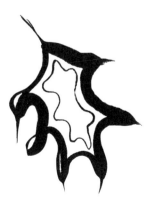

*Monk: What will happen when the leaves fall
and the trees are bare?*

Unmon: The Golden Wind.

HEGIKAN ROKU

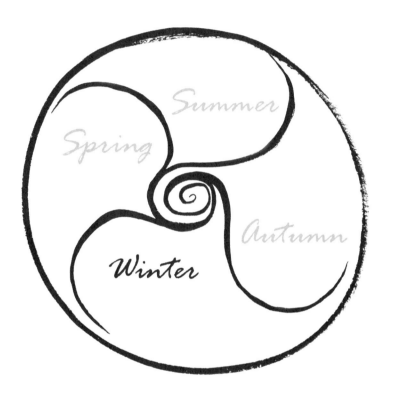

first snow

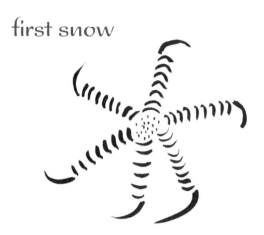

outside

slowly taking one step after another
wait for the breath and the movement to harmonise …

look around, and smile …
let the smile spread everywhere …

breathe in through the left foot which is light
and breathe out through the right foot which is heavy …
light – heavy, light – heavy

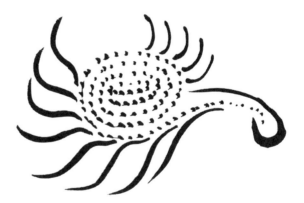

standing

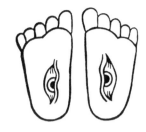

feel the feet well-supported by the ground,
join the hands in front of the heart ...

facing east
inhale and exhale sounding a prolonged 'A'
several times ...

facing south
extend the toes ...
inhale and exhale sounding a prolonged 'U'
the rhythm of the breath is natural,
with no strain or effort ...
several times ...

facing west
the contact with the ground gives stability
and lets the spine extend towards the sky ...
inhale and exhale with the sound 'M'
several times ...

facing north
inhale and exhale prolonging the sound 'AUM'
several times ...

release the arms
lengthen forward
the dorsal spine extends
feel the base of the skull moving further away
from the tailbone ...
return to upright with full awareness
letting the knees slightly bend
and the heels sink into the ground

bring the hands together behind the back ...
the elbows relaxed, the wrists touching ...
the little fingers in contact and resting on the space
between the shoulder blades ...

exhale towards the ground,
inhale,
the area of the heart opens with a smile

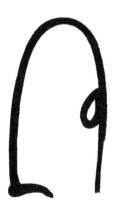

unwinding the spine

bring attention into the heels …
the toes extend and separate …
feel the flexibility in the ankles …
exhale and lengthen forwards
following the rhythm of the breath …

repeat on the other side
calmly …

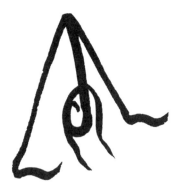

take the feet further apart …
feel the connection between the tailbone and heels …
exhaling …
lengthen forwards …
let the arms go …
inhale and exhale in this new space …

sitting on the heels

let the forehead move towards the ground ...
the arms extend beyond the head ...

through the legs which rest on the ground
let go of all the weight and the weariness in the body ...

through the forehead let go of all the noise,
any thoughts and worries ...

through the palms of the hands on the ground
release any troubling emotions and their heaviness ...

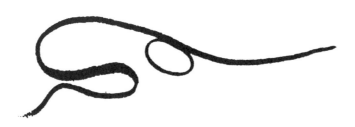

place the hands on the ground beside the head …
like two big ears …
lift the pelvis …
let the top of the head rest on the ground
inhale and exhale …
letting the back of the neck soften and extend
so the space between the cervical vertebrae expands
inhale and exhale …

return to a sitting position

put the hands on the sacrum … interweave the fingers …
lift the pelvis again …
the top of the head touches the ground …
inhale and exhale
letting the arms straighten and move up …
feel them lengthening … towards the sky
with an exhalation bring the spine to upright

listen …

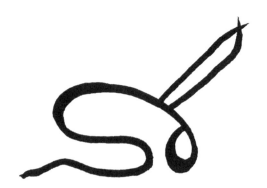

exhaling, the right arm lengthens and extends
and wraps around the back …
the back of the hand in contact with the body
the left hand resting on the opposite knee …
inhale and exhale …
release the stretch …
bring attention back to the spine

repeat on the other side …

change the position of the legs,
sit with the legs crossed …
place the hands below the navel …
inhale through the nose
and exhale sounding 'AUM' for several minutes

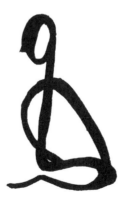

deep relaxation

rest on your back with arms and feet spread wide apart
like a peaceful starfish on the sandy bottom of the sea

visualise the navel and the area behind the navel
let wider and wider circles swirl out from that centre
towards the extreme periphery of your being ...
as far as the tips of your fingers, as far as the tips of your toes
let the palms of the hands relax
let the soles of the feet relax
let the breath be naturally curious to reach the tips of the fingers
and the tips of the toes from within
let the breath become deep and rhythmical, like the waves of the ocean
flowing in and out
soothing
deeply refreshing and cleansing

feel the ground actively absorbing any sediment of tiredness
the pores of the skin have released
let your body return to a state of innocence and peace

let yourself be empty, completely empty
let the next exhalation travel through empty space within
until it touches the soles of the feet
relax and let the body sink into the earth
inhale slowly
repeat this journey a few times

in the depth of winter

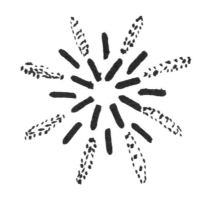

standing

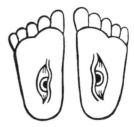

let the toes get longer
growing out from the centre of the feet ...
make space between the toes ...
sense the shape, and the impression the footprint makes on the ground

take a step forward ...
find the solidity of the base again ...
the feet implant a sense of stability ...
inhaling bring the arms up ...
exhaling let them spread out, and then fly above the head ...
there is a sense of lightness in the upper part of the body ...
the arms spread out and lift like great wings ...

bring the feet close to each other again, parallel,
  then take a step forward with the other foot ...

experiment with this position
  with the forward knee straight and then slightly bent ...
  let the body enjoy the natural elongation that follows
  breathe ...

feel the wave ...

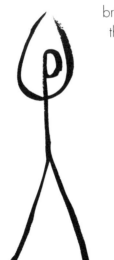

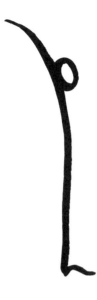

then move close to a wall …
keep the feet even with each other,
the great toes facing forward
give them a precise direction …
breathe in and out
let the arms rise up …
let the body lengthen so the fingers almost brush against the ceiling …

feel the wave …

then lengthen forwards to rest the spine …
repeat this movement several times
letting the body explore the space within,
and around, and above …
feel its entire length …
and with this practice encourage each vertebra
to find more space
a greater distance from the others …
to create new spaces which spread,
and lengthen, and expand
receiving nourishment from the air

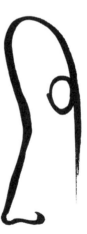

stretched out on the ground

hug the knees,
sense the shape of the sacrum touching the ground …
let the arms stay long by the sides of the body then
exhale and bring awareness to the shoulders,
while the shoulders are opening towards the ground,
simultaneously extend the wrists …

listening to the breath for a few minutes
prepare the position with great tranquillity

exhaling bring the legs above the head …
the rhythm of the breath changes,
but check to be sure it is always supple and flowing …
occasionally with an exhalation lengthen the heels
and sense how this movement makes the pelvis
more lively, more light …

let one leg come up
and then the other
finally both legs …

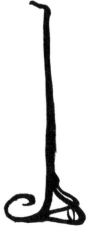

bring the arms behind the head,
with the hands take hold of the feet or the ankles
and start to slowly come down
accompanying the movement with the breath …

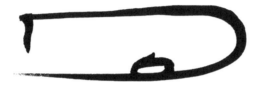

repeat the position, calmly …
when the feet are behind the head
use tiny steps to take them further apart
the spine is pleased to get longer …
trust the contact the shoulders make with the ground …
how reassuring …
see how gradually the legs and body can come down

breathe …
let the exhalation become long and deep

winter is silent

sitting with crossed legs ...
the base of the body settles down
the position becomes comfortable and stable ...
release any tightness in the shoulders, or the jaw ...
exhaling, bring the hands in front of the body ...
put the pads of the tips of the little fingers together
and the ring fingers ...

breathe for a few minutes
keeping this contact,
and then change to let the pads of the middle fingers touch
and release the contact with the other fingers for a few minutes
sensing the changes this brings ...
then shift the points of contact to the index fingers and the thumbs
something is still changing
while the breath is flowing in and out

then let the tips of all five fingers on one hand
meet the tips of the fingers on the other ...
maintain this contact
listening to the rhythm of the breath ...

let the hands rest on the legs,
stretch out on the ground later

icy cold

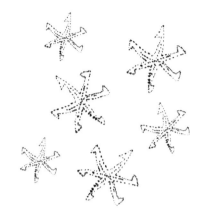

standing

breathing, bring awareness to the position of the body …
let the feet settle on the ground,
give attention to the ankles …
explore the shape of the ankles
and the shape of the space between the two of them …
with the exhalation the heels press lightly
down into the ground …
and release with the inhalation …

imagine that the heels are extending far away
from the toes and with the next exhalation
they sink into the ground …
with an inhalation the feet are big and stable …

turn the right foot towards the outside
and the left towards the inside …
wait for the position to become
calm and still …

in the exhalation
find the contact with the ground again,
in the inhalation
the lightness in the arms
which lengthen further away
from the upper back …

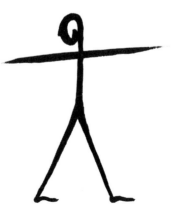

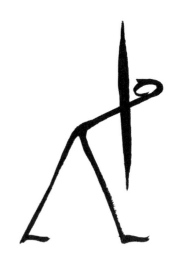

turn the head towards the left shoulder
and wait to feel stable from the waist down,
and light from the waist up …
go back to the position with the feet together,
listen to the breath for a few minutes
then repeat on the other side …

go back to the centre, and this time,
turning the feet as before,
when the back heel is planted firmly
lengthen from that heel to the tips of the fingers …

look towards the opposite shoulder …
breathing …
but before going down
let the shoulders become level and in line with the feet
and for the shoulders to feel light …
then lengthen out and down
letting the spine release,
with the breath …

repeat on the other side …
then lengthen forwards,
letting the spine unfurl

bring the arms above the head,
with elbows slightly bent ...

breathing, sense the feet growing roots
and the upper part of the body
becoming light ...

getting longer ...

it is an invitation to bend backwards
without effort

stay and play with the wave created
by exhaling into the roots
releasing everything down

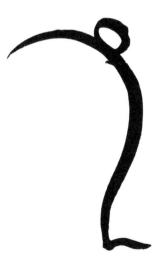

stretch out on the ground

with the knees bent …
exhaling, sense the contact between the feet and the ground increasing …
inhaling, place the attention on the upper back …
on its desire to get longer …
and slowly slowly let the sacrum rise from the floor …
while the shoulders and head rest on the ground …

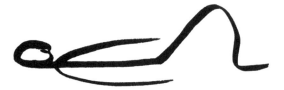

let the sacrum return to the ground,
hold onto the knees …
feel the breath is moving through the body like a wave …
washing away tension …
releasing old knots and snarls …
the wave becomes so powerful,
it turns into movement …
feel how the body lengthens
naturally in this position …

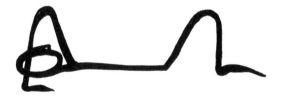

place the hands beside the head …
until …
the body comes up without any effort …
with a great deal of space around the waist …
the body is like a light bow or arch …
gently let the body return to the ground …
put the hands on the insides of the knees
hug them …
continue breathing …

repeat this movement several times
letting it become more enjoyable …
more fluid, more ample …

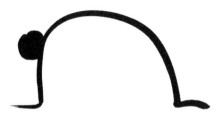

sitting with the legs straight

the feet close to each other…
exhaling, sense the way the sitting bones
contact the ground …
this helps the energy bounce upwards …

let the spine transmit this movement …
the part of the body touching the ground is heavy …
an invitation rises out of the ground …
the arms move

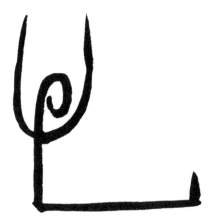

this movement helps feel the lightness
throughout the length of the spine …
exhaling, bring the arms down towards the ground …
from the pelvis lengthen forwards …

gradually with the breath lengthening forwards
with the neck in line with the sacrum …
the upper back dances between these two places …

this position takes time …

breathe …

listen …

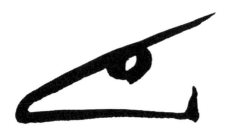

the breath that brings clarity

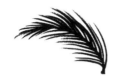

sitting with the legs crossed place one hand on the sacrum
and the other low on the abdomen…
listen to the breath in the space between the hands …

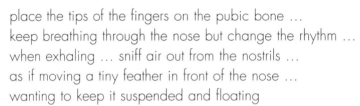

place the tips of the fingers on the pubic bone …
keep breathing through the nose but change the rhythm …
when exhaling … sniff air out from the nostrils …
as if moving a tiny feather in front of the nose …
wanting to keep it suspended and floating

experiment with this rhythm …
make a pause often
to inhale and exhale naturally
to feel the quality of the space
created by this new 'teacher' …

check to be sure the mouth is relaxed
the shoulders resting calmly
and the pulsation keeps going deeper down

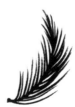

stretch out on the ground …
and enjoy the silence and the space
created by the practice

winter relaxation

stretch out on the ground,
begin to follow a path
to the interior of the body

bring the attention within,
moving from the crown of the head towards the feet …
pausing along the central line of the body …
feel a smile is spreading behind the eyes
illuminating the inside of the head

let the attention sink down into the chest
and feel how the area behind the breastbone around the heart
can expand in a smile …

slowly shift attention behind the navel
and let a smile blossom there …

a mountain grove, leafless –
cloudless skies, windstill —
dawn colours pinch the frost; chill moonlight overflows.
all Heaven and Earth should bear the name-board
'Palace of Broad Cold'.

KOKAN SHIREN

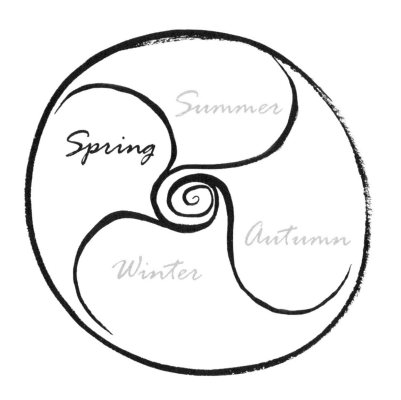

scattered showers

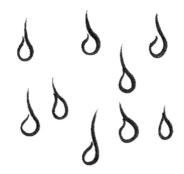

in the open air

walk slowly, slowly,
until a regular rhythm emerges …
inhale and take three steps,
exhale and take three steps …

the heel meets the ground
the sole of the foot spreads out happily …

a rhythm takes over
walking becomes light and lilting …
steps fall like rain drops

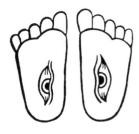

standing

notice the shape of the feet settled on the ground …
bring attention and weight into the right foot …
listening for any changes …
bring attention and weight into the left foot …
inhale, exhale, listen …
repeating several times …
at the end of the exhalation the foot plants itself fully down,
and grows roots …

the base becomes broader and more stable
draw the hands together in front of the heart,
the chin turns to the left …
the right foot settles into the ground …
sends down thick roots …
the chin turns to the right …
the left foot settles into the ground …
and puts down strong big roots

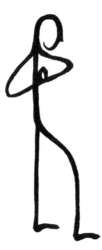

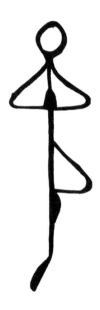

the attention stays on the right foot on the ground
while bringing the sole of the other foot
to the inside of the thigh …
again hands join together in front of the heart …
breathe …

let the hands rise up …
feel like a tree sustained by its roots
and drawing up,
towards the light …

standing,
find the position again …
the breath …

then repeat on the other side

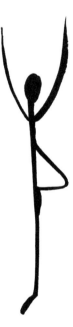

take a small step forward
and bend the knee
without losing the weight
in the heel behind …

with hands together
in front of the heart,
exhale
and shift the weight forwards …
the leg behind lifts,
the arms fly beyond the head …
roots are growing deeper …
under the foot on the ground …

then give just as much time and attention
to the other side

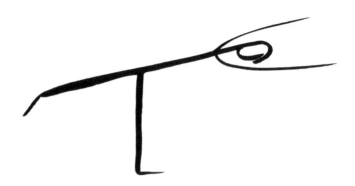

lying on the back

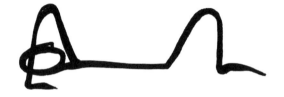

with knees bent …
the spinal column gets longer …
exhale towards the feet
and notice whether they open simultaneously …
wait until this happens …

bring the hands to the side of the head,
exhaling, the heels sink into the ground …
the upper back unrolls, the pelvis lifts …

hands and feet continue to open
to the contact with the ground,
the tailbone keeps lengthening …
come up with an exhalation
and feel that the hands and feet
are smiling and spreading

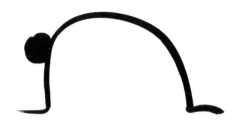

on the back holding the knees

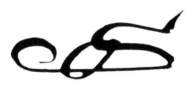

perhaps a yawn comes …

place the hands and feet on the ground …
there is a widening smile in the centre of the hands and feet …
yawning …

let the spine get longer
and let the pelvis come up
so now it is suspended …
with the help of an exhalation

when the spine slowly returns to the ground
let the nape of the neck find its connection with the sacrum …
let the legs get longer …
yawning …
let a stretch grow from one hand
towards the opposite foot …

repeat several times

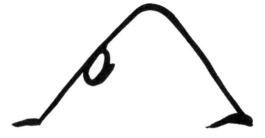

sitting on the ground

prepare the legs for half lotus position
listen to the breathing …
find the 'breath that brings clarity' again,
a great 'instructor' able to show
the way into the position …

the upper back responds to this breath
and links the ground with the sky …
giving a sense of trust and cleansing

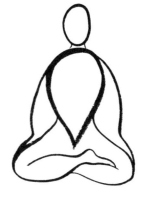

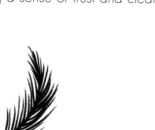

the rousing of the insects

breathing like a bumble bee

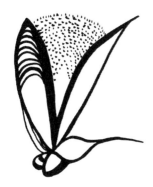

gravity gives a way to find
roots and alignment

while standing
inhale through the nostrils,
and exhale through almost closed lips
imitating the buzz of an insect ...

lips are softly parted ...
they vibrate during the exhalation ...
playing with this sound ...
until a rhythm comes into play ...
spending a few minutes with no sense of hurry ...
then start to breathe silently again ...

listen to the cadence of the exhalation, inhalation ...
and then ...
return to the sound of the buzzing bee,
letting it vibrate along each vertebra ...
while the feet get bigger ...
the arms rise over the head, lightly ...
keep playing with the vibrating breath ...

lengthen forwards …
the spine rests in this position …
the weight of the head lets the neck and
body find their length

pay attention to the toes
without letting them curl
or fill with weight …
all the back of the body gets longer …
experiment with prolonging the exhalation
and let the heels sink into the ground …
the knees are not tight …
and with this movement let the body come up again …

give time to this sequence:
lengthen forward with the head heavy and low
letting the entire spinal column roll down
and then roll up again with the head trailing
until it becomes easy, fluid …
so the whole body
is fully aware

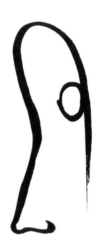

sitting on the heels

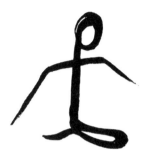

find a large and stable base again
check to be sure it is comfortable
(pillows can be a help) …
feel the reverberation of the 'buzzing bumble bee'
all along the spine …
almost a massage,
subtle, profound …

place the hands on the ground behind the feet
and let the legs get lighter,
ease the ankles, and feet
with little circular movements …

return to the knees,
feel the force of gravity
and the way it anchors the pelvis …
the sacrum is drawn downwards …
play a bit with the arms
letting them come up …
with elbows slightly bent …

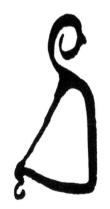

exhale and bring the hands onto the heels …
the upper back gets longer

exhaling, the right arm lengthens and extends …
it wraps behind the body …
the back of the hand in contact with the body
the left hand resting on the opposite knee …
inhale and exhale …
release tensions …
bring the attention back to the spine …

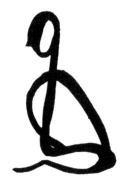

then repeat on the other side …

change the position of the legs
and sit with crossed legs …
bring the hands below the navel …
and inhale through the nose
and exhale through the nose
for several minutes

sitting

with the legs spread wide …
massage the backs of the knees

inhale,
the arms rise up,
exhale and let the weight of the pelvis
and the sacrum sink down into the ground …

turn and look at the left foot,
let the body extend out along the left leg …
exhale …
all the left side of the body releases …
repeat on the other side …
looking towards the horizon, far away …

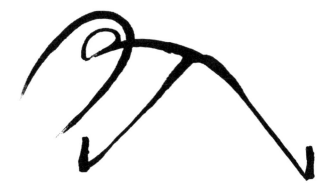

lie on the ground …
the knees are bent …
let the sound of the 'buzzing bumble bee'
go down the upper back
dissolving knots, grooming tangles,
removing tiredness,
until it reaches the sacrum …
give time to this practice …

… return to silent breathing
and slowly release the legs

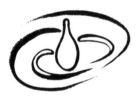

pure light

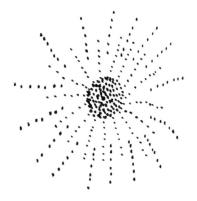

swinging

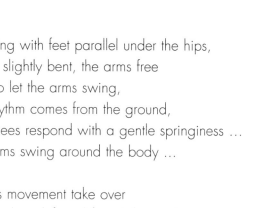

standing with feet parallel under the hips,
knees slightly bent, the arms free
start to let the arms swing,
the rhythm comes from the ground,
the knees respond with a gentle springiness …
the arms swing around the body …

let this movement take over
from right to left and from left to right …
the eyes are open and follow the movement …

the movement slowly comes to an end …

return to the centre,
place the hands below the navel and listen …

    listen to the breath and feel how the gravity is active,
    it is present in the feet, legs, pelvis …

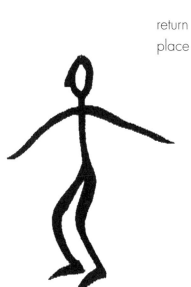

turn the right foot out …
feel the heel is firmly grounded,
shift the weight to this foot
and the front knee bends …

with an inhalation let the arms
come up without any effort …
the elbows slightly bent …
exhale and the arms go down …

inhale and the arms come up …
they extend like wings …
they float on the air …

the eyes trace
the entire length of the arms …
first looking at the hand behind …
when there is stability pause
looking at the hand in front …
give the same attention to the other side …

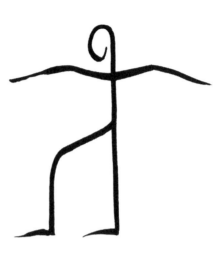

repeat the preceding sequence
with a greater distance between the feet ...
the back heel sinks into the ground
and the upper back gets longer ...
the top of the head is drawn towards the sky ...

breathe for some time in this position ...
gradually extend, letting the spine lengthen out of the hips
until the right hand touches the ground ...
the roots under the feet are thick and strong ...

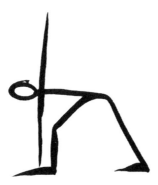

give the other side the same attention ...
without any hurry ...
with the attention on the breath going out,
the breath coming in

lying on the front

breathing smoothly, let the ground absorb any resistance
bring the hands to the sides of the chest …
the elbows move closer together with an exhalation
and move apart with an inhalation …
rest the forehead on the ground
release the vertebrae in the neck …
exposing the occipital area to the light …
exhale with a syllable… SSS …
and come up in the cobra position …

the upper back sparkles with vitality …

repeat several times
resting on the ground between each …
gravity makes the legs heavy on the ground

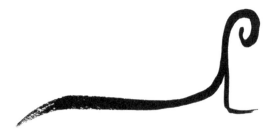

four legged

let the hands and feet open ...

while exhaling
let the entire length of the spine
and the legs lengthen ...
then return on the heels ...

repeat ...
exhaling towards hands and feet

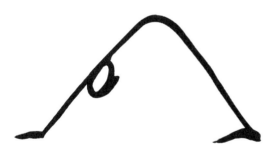

the resting Buddha

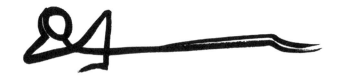

lie on the back with the knees bent,
extending an arm above the head …
exhale, and lengthen the leg on that side …
feel a lengthening from the waist towards the soles of the feet
and towards the palms of the hands …

notice how the exhalation
encourages this double movement …

turn on this side …
gravity is very powerful …
letting go
and feeling the contact of this side with the ground …

wait for the position to become comfortable and silent …
bend the elbow
resting the neck in the palm of the hand …
any tightness in the armpit smoothes out, the neck relaxes …

the eyes rest behind slightly closed lids
not looking for details, but gazing peacefully …

inhale and exhale
until there is a state of profound repose …

spring relaxation

spread out with the back on the ground,
feel how the exhalation
lets the body settle more fully on the ground …
listen to the sound of the air as it leaves the nostrils …
listen to the sound of the air as it comes into the nostrils …
the air that goes out takes away many impurities …
the air that comes in is enriching, nourishing …

keep the attention on the passage of the air
through the nostrils for a few minutes …

now draw attention to the lungs,
within the rib cage …
the breath is natural …
without effort …
feel how the lungs slowly empty …
and feel how gradually
they open to receive new air

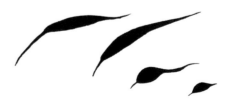

of the ten thousand trees
along the banks of the river
the apricots have just come into flower
in the wind of a night

WANG WEI

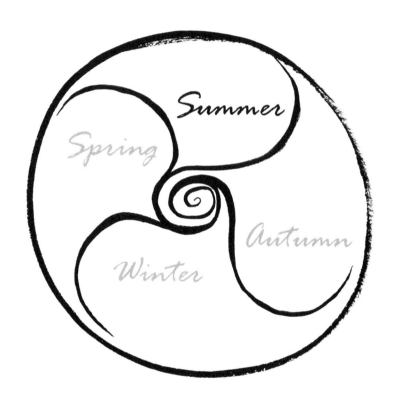

tassels of corn

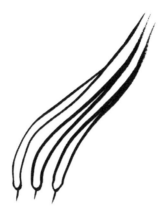

in the open air

with short steps ...
exhale through the feet into the ground,
inhale through the feet up from the ground ...
exhale into the ground, inhale from the ground ...

this awareness and contact with the earth brings calm ...
the feet expand and revive ...
walk in this way for a few minutes

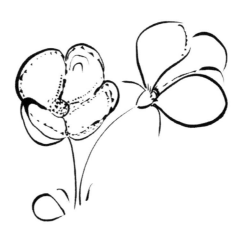

sitting

with the legs long and space between them …
let the weight sink into the pelvis
and the hands run along the parts of the legs
that touch the ground …

coaxing them to drop and let go …
pause at the skin behind the knees
wait for this space to soften
so intimate and contained …

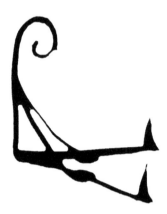

bend the knees
and put the soles of the feet together ...

with an inhalation the arms rise up
and the hands join above the head ...
exhale and the hands come down ...
the hands pause above the head,
rest for a few breaths ...

the hands joined together move down in front
of the face and stop there for a few breaths,
then they go down in front of the heart
and pause there for several breaths ...

paying attention to the rhythm of the breathing ...
repeat several times slowly,
with awareness ...

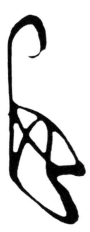

extend the right leg,
the left hand goes towards the right foot,
if this feels awkward
the hand can rest on the outside of the knee,
exhale, the spine becomes free
and can lean forward without effort,
feeling the neck always in line with the sacrum …
the back of the waist expands and extends …
sense the movements in the upper back …
the more it is free the more the body can go forwards …

repeat calmly
on the other side …

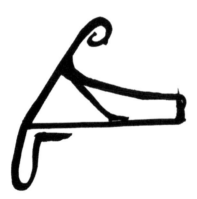

from this position,
grow deep roots from the waist down ...
wait for the body to become very silent ...
the elbows slightly bent ...
the upper back becomes a link
between heaven and earth ...

breathe ...
pay attention for a movement from within

let the spine slowly come back to vertical,
keeping its soft curves,
its natural flexibility ...

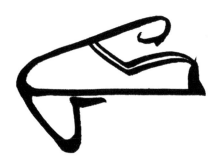

sitting between the heels

with a pillow between the heels …
gently rotate the calves towards the outside …
the side of the foot gets longer …
the big toes face each other …
it helps to give the little toes a tug
gradually settle down and sit between the feet …

breathe until the position becomes comfortable …
and the base broad and heavy …
release the legs …

repeat the movement of the arms
used at the beginning of the practice …
pause with the hands joined above the head …
let them go down in front of the face …
then in front of the heart …

on hands and knees

with the hands well planted on the ground
play with the breath and the back ...
let the weight go down towards the ground
through the hands, knees and feet ...

shift the weight from the hands to the knees ...
stretch the body encouraged by gravity ...
until ...
the sacrum rises,
the legs straighten,
the hands and feet spread
opening from the centre

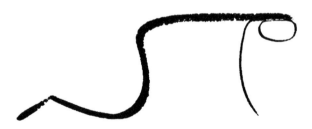

the breath that takes me home

sitting on the heels,
wait for the position to become easy,
without any hurry,
release the shoulders,
leave space between the two rows of teeth,
a space that relaxes
and softens the neck ... become aware
of how the upper back is lengthening and releasing ...
breathe ...
and through the spine connect again
with the ground below the feet and the sky above the head ...
exhale through the mouth
as if pronouncing a silent 'A'
and let the chin go further down ...
let anything that is heavy, tired, dusty
seep away ...

inhale through the nose
bringing the head into line
with the rest of the upper back ...

let this movement become more fluid
and in time with the rhythm of the breath,
give a few minutes to this practice

great heat

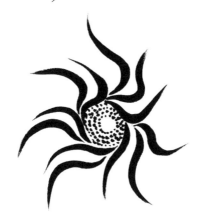

spread out on the back

close to a wall, with the bottom against the wall
and the legs resting long and straight along the wall,
let them empty,
let their weight go down into the ground …
the pelvis, back and the head are resting …
let the little knots in the neck release and
wrap the arms across the front of the body
to hold the backs of the shoulders …

bend the knees and put the soles of the feet together …
give attention to the force of gravity …
bring the arms up …
then above the head … exhaling

with the right hand hold the left wrist,
and gently roll it towards the sky …
feel how this movement travels towards the hip …
repeat with the other hand …

change the position of the legs:
let them extend and spread wide against the wall …
let the wall support them …

bring the palms
of the hands to face upwards …
rest the shoulders on the ground
the arms become silent …

bend the knees
and place the soles
of the feet on the wall …
exhale towards the wrists …
shoulders, arms, elbows,
wrists and hands finally
touch the ground …

with tiny steps climb up the wall
resting the soles of the feet firmly …
lift the sacrum …
the knees stay bent …
take several breaths …

use little steps to go back to the ground
letting the spine settle down one vertebra at a time …
repeat until the movement becomes easy …

breathing feel the base of support
formed by the shoulders and elbows …
relax the throat, the chin …
feel the contact between the ground and the neck
dissolving clogged energy …
take one foot away from the wall, then the other …

repeat the positions of the legs
that were practiced before on the wall …
first with the legs close to each other …
then spread apart …
then bending the knees
and bringing the soles of the feet together …
pause and breathe during each of them …

rest the feet on the wall,
making contact …
and with the knees bent
move down the wall slowly with little steps

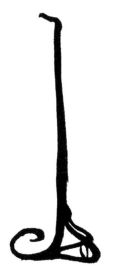

spread out on the ground with the knees bent ...
resting the hands by the side of the sternum ...

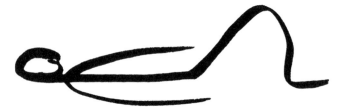

probing the area around the collarbone with finger tips
to create more space ...
space for the passage of air ...

inhaling ...
exhaling ...
invite a smile ...

the refreshing breath

sitting on the heels …
inhale slowly 'sucking' the air through the lips,
the chin rises up,
the shoulders stay calm …
exhale, the chin slowly goes down towards the sternum …

for a few minutes …
curl the sides of the tongue delicately …
suck the air as if through a straw …
the tongue curls …
like a leaf which lets fresh water drain …
the chin goes up …
exhale through the lips while the chin goes down …
the back of the neck gets longer …
the movement is soft, rhythmic, like the breath

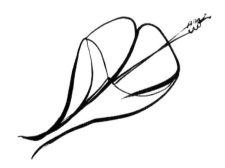

summer wanes

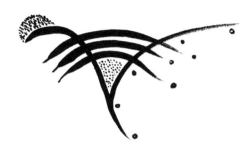

on the ground

close the eyes …
the lids are light as leaves floating on water …
the eyes rest …
gently place the base of the hands on the cheeks
and the base of the fingers on the eyebrows
so that the eyes are enclosed in a space
that is dark and friendly …
the eyes feel protected by this darkness …
they slide into a space in the head …
where they can rest …

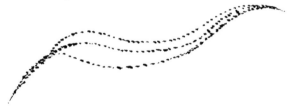

let light filter through the spaces
between the fingers waiting to open …
the eyes receive the increase of light
while the arms rest on the ground …
slowly open the eyes again,
blinking,
with the refreshing rest
colours are brighter colours

hold the knees
the spine lets all tension go into the ground …

extend one leg
and then the other, upwards …
without effort
let the feet, ankles, knees empty

shake them a bit to help them fully relax …
let the arms go up
and shake them gently
feel them emptying and becoming lighter …

then bend the knees
take hold of one
with an exhalation let the other lengthen close to the ground
and let it swing
let it rest
until the ground makes it heavy …

repeat on the other side

sitting

with the soles of the feet together
close to the body
inhale
and let the knees
come up without effort …
breathe
and let the knees go down as much as they would like …

repeat the movement several times,
until the tensions in the legs relax …

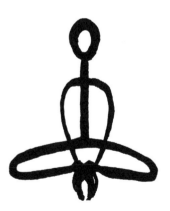

extend the legs parallel
the wrists resting on the ground at the sides of the pelvis …
exhale and extend the heels …
inhale and expand …
exhale and open the wrists towards the ground …
become aware of a small natural pause …
inhale, and feel the space
that fills with new air

with the legs long, open them as wide as comfortable …
the exhalation releases the sacrum towards the ground
and lets the body bend forward …
lengthen according to the breath …
the spine dances

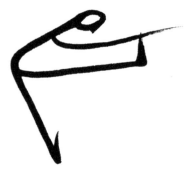

sitting between the heels

with a pillow between the heels …
gently turn the flesh of the calves outwards …
the sides of the feet lengthen …
the big toes face each other …
gradually settle down
and sit between the feet …

breathe until the position becomes comfortable …
and the base broad and heavy

then release the legs

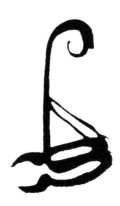

stretch out on the ground

on one side with the knees bent …
the arms extended
with the hands together …
very slowly while exhaling,
the hand above slides beyond the other hand …
then it retracts until the hand moves across the chest …
and the arm extends on the other side …
breathe for some while

enjoy the openness of this position …

repeat until the breath
and the movement harmonise …

turn on the opposite side

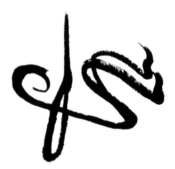

sitting

with crossed legs …
let the base become broad and easy …
so the upper back can feel free to
release, to lengthen …

repeat the refreshing breathing
exhaling this time through the nose …
taste the freshness, the calm,
the ease

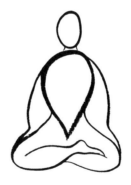

summer relaxation

stretch out on the ground,
giving attention to the shape of the bones of the skull …
shift attention to the bones of the right arm
and how long they are …
then on the bones of the left arm …
and how long they are …

explore the shape of the upper back …
become aware of the vertebra, one after another,
count them slowly starting with the nape of the neck
and going down towards the coccyx …
become aware of the beauty of the whole back
and on the hollow places within the spine …

draw attention down along the bones of the right leg
and discover their shape …
ending with the right foot …
go down along the bones of the left leg
and discover their shape …
ending with the left foot …

feel all the bones of the body resting on the ground,
and finding their natural alignment,
and how this contact with the ground revitalises them

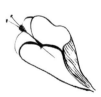

put all your attention into the nerve,
delicate as the stele of a lotus,
in the centre of your upper back
transform yourself into that

DIALOGUE BETWEEN SHIVA AND DEVI

in the cycle of seasons: reflections

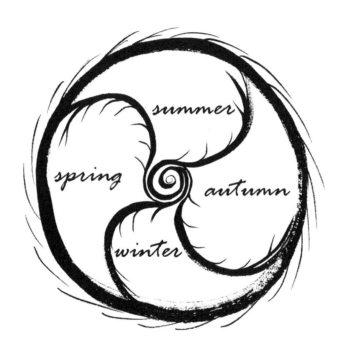

I let myself be blown by the wind
East and West
like a fallen leaf or a dry pot
and I cannot say whether the wind is riding me
or I am riding the wind

FROM THE BOOK OF LAO TZU

Autumn stimulates a new and familiar rhythm. The weather, and changes in nature, the return to the patterns of daily life all encourage us to reflect and to slow down. The leaves which once gleamed with light and swayed with any breeze, now are chastened by wind and rain. Eventually they fall, darken and dry up. They appear withered and lifeless, although this may actually be their way to offer space for a different rhythm. Detachment, loss, withdrawal are the characteristics which define the autumnal phase[4].

Tuning into this change is a sort of landscape maintenance, pruning branches that are no longer useful and letting the leaves fall. Through practice we acquire the capacity to savour autumn colours.

Walking practice helps listen to the rustle of dry leaves, which are not yet part of the earth but are down waiting for water to help them be absorbed and transformed. Slow steps bring harmony with the particular signs of autumn and the woods with their various colours, the sounds in the air.

The days shorten, a tinge of melancholy enters, the rhythm changes, the celebrations of summer are over, the light and heat have subsided. We move towards something mellow and soft, which encourages us to look within and to reflect …

This becomes a journey inwards to set 'the house' in order, using ancient rituals like sorting the drawers and cupboards, cleaning the cellar, throwing out old things, to ready the internal space for the possibilities of the coming season. Autumn is a time to adopt many different breathing rhythms …

Breath is the key element, in autumn and in spring, seasons of transition; traditionally in India pranayama was taught in these two seasons. It offers crucial assistance through phases of transformation, calling for more commitment, more participation, a keener sense of readiness.

The practice can include a series of small movements which help us to perceive the space of the breath, and become more aware of its range and rhythm.

To contact the richness of the season, its various ways of letting things go … to open the window and to look out and welcome the elements nature offers us – the sounds of the leaves when we walk or how they float through the air and rest on the ground, also the darkness and tediousness of rainy days and the special atmosphere of mist and fog … yoga practice offers a way to welcome all these elements and learn how to savour their special subtlety.

Bow to the trees,
Bow to the leaves –
Autumn lessons

Autumn is the season in which we gather fruit with a strong skin, or nuts with a hard shell like chestnuts, walnuts, hazelnuts, with their richness within, compact and intensely nourishing. We feel inclined to get in contact with the inner part inside the shell, our deeper, vital parts, and sense a need for moving within, and letting the pace slow down … to create a structure, with a solid boundary which is also permeable and lets us communicate. This is the time schools start again, plans, telephone calls, meetings … communication. A tinge of sadness can arise, like a mist, which lifts before it disperses …

In winter the seed is waiting underground: nothing seems to be happening, but this waiting holds its entire potential.

There is silence. The damp earth under the snow. The vital energy retracts below, listening.

It is the same quality we find in the little pause at the end of the exhalation, that pause before the breath changes direction and the exhalation transforms itself into a new inhalation. A pause which has a resting, listening, silent presence. This is winter, with the bare trees showing the shape of the branches, their structure, waiting for messages to come from the earth and the sky, stimulation to grow new buds and start a new cycle.

Being in harmony means to give time for these pauses of listening, to become aware of our framework: the alignment of the bones, the lengthening of the deep layers of muscles and the tissues that wrap our densest, bony parts. To recognise and to sense the vitality of our bony structure, and allow the waters within us to flow and nourish and revive this structure.

The seed deep in the dark earth lives in a dreamy state of sleep. To listen means also to get in touch with our unconscious, a world submerged, and to grant it space, not to compress or suffocate it with excessive activity. To recognise and accept a slow pulse which speaks to us of our needs in order to begin a new cycle with greater lightness, cleansed and bathed by the limpid waters from our greatest depths.

Attending to the calm of winter cultivates the internal fire. The practice nourishes this fire under the embers, the flame that helps keep the river of life flowing. Standing positions in winter emphasise our roots and help keep us warm. When we repeat them often, they reveal their depths. They help us to adjust with the cold climate, and avoid sliding into any torpor.

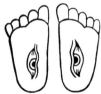

Outdoors, by the sea or in the mountains we sense the energy present in the air, prana, and nourish ourselves with its special quality, rendered terse and vibrant by a long journey across the sea, through scented forests, enriched by the sun and wind and the mysterious movements of earth, sun and stars …

Perhaps this is what we feel we often miss in the winter, spending much of the time indoors, forced to breathe poor air which weakens us. The reluctance to stay outdoors for long becomes a habit; we tuck ourselves in, make a nest, and this makes us more lazy.

As soon as the sun comes out we can go outside and start to walk slowly, listening, finding that precious contact with the ground again.

In the winter the seed lies dormant, and the positions tend to crystallise. In the spring we want to try something new. We experience familiar positions with a fresh rhythm and find them renewed, more intelligent, more vivid and more interesting, as if the winter had transformed them and let them grow.

From one day to the next the light changes, and gradually increases. We can respond to this light, and the flowering, budding and growing in an individual way with our practice. A new phase of adaptation and experiment lets this energy flow through us.

Winds are cold and biting, which we find bracing but also hard to bear. Wind is unsettling, and makes us fragile. Just as we are getting used to the silent rhythm of winter, spring seems to tap us on the shoulder and urge us to wake up.

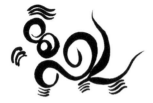

Dear flat rock
    facing the stream
Where the willows are sweeping
    over my wine cup again
If you say that the spring wind
    has no understanding
Why should it come blowing me
    these falling flowers?   **WANG WEI**

Spring brings spurts of excitement and deep restlessness: the buds grow silently while for human beings the spring is noisy. We are full of plans and projects, sometimes sensible, sometimes raving. We expect wonderful marvellous things to happen and if they don't we feel very disappointed. We sway from one mood to its opposite.

'The mysterious powers of the spring create the wind.' The wind blows, disturbing our vision, burning our eyes. It raises dust. Energy is not smooth, it's full of jerks. It sparkles, it is effervescent. We stumble as if hitting against invisible barriers that try to curb its overwhelming nature. When it finds space it start to flow again.

This tends to upset the liver, that great metabolising organ which needs to be healthy. Spring is its special moment. The liver brings the vision of dawn, the great horizon, the direction so we can organise life without feeling overwhelmed by it. It is a metaphysical as well as a physical organ: it is a wonderful metabolic lab with five hundred different functions and a powerful filter, which needs to rest at night.

Spring brings out excitement and wonder, and the practice modulates the jangle of its extremes. We introduce twists to promote flexibility: we consider the sides as well as the front and back of the body, like a rushing stream which needs clean banks. We feel the need to get longer again: in the winter the mists, the clouds and the sky have let us fold in on ourselves; in spring we feel a great desire to look around and expand.

Yoga positions help us discover the polarity between the earth and the sky again, where the sky becomes more distant and the flowers, grass, and especially the trees remind us of this movement up from below. The earth holds such vital force, which finds expression through the buds, emerging leaves, new growth. We need to find access to this swirling energy through our practice.

Balancing postures with the eyes open strengthen our vision, while the roots acquire greater stability, and help us stay alert to changes.
The quality of presence encourages fluidity and suppleness, rather than rigidity …

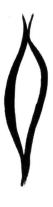

Summer is the season of completeness … when all the flaking and fragmenting we have experienced in the other seasons come together again. Summer brings a sense of fullness … The days become so much brighter and longer, and the sun is stronger. Perhaps this offers us the feeling of 'having arrived', because the light is at its greatest splendour. The vision and the capacity to focus, which gave so many problems in the springtime, seem more clear in the summer …

If we harmonise with the incoming season, it will let us accomplish what we had only glimpsed before. Spring is like a tiring journey, with stops and starts, forward and backward and zigzag. A tumultuous process. With the arrival of summer, we feel we have reached a place where it is possible to enjoy a sense of completeness. The positions on the floor help us explore the possibilities of this transition, and this sense of completeness.

Finally we can expose our body to light and warmth, shedding many things, baring ourselves, and covering ourselves now with colours. The smiles of spring have turned into a more diffuse joy, it feels good to offer the body to light, and our smile can even expand into a laugh.

When the sun becomes too intrusively strong, fixed in the sky, we need to offset this with shelter, and find shady places. Practice refreshes, and brings refuge, where we can withdraw from the dazzling sun.

Just a hint of thunder clouds
in the evening sky.
On summer mountains,
the faint disk of the moon —
night just beginning.   SOGI

Summer storms come with roaring thunder and streaks of lightning. They clear the air after so much heat and stagnation. Storms are dramatic and the body doesn't know how to interpret such violence and huddles until the storm clears. Then the body can release its fears and tensions. School ends in the summer and brings a sense of liberty, a chance to play and be free, to reinvent oneself. This sense of play and memories of sand and sea water encourage us to become children again and let our dreams flower. This makes the cycle complete.

It may be hard to say goodbye to summer when autumn is in the air, and to welcome the changes after such dazzle. The practice helps us. It offers an invitation to become smaller again, and content when the skies are less bright. Sometimes the end of summer may bring a sense of relief at the change of pace, the ending of the hot spell, all the activities and celebrations. We sense that life has been pleasant but superficial ... so we wish to return to school, to regain our roots. The practice helps us, it is an invitation to become smaller again, and be happy when the skies are less bright.

Often we move in a dimension we like which is also quite superficial ... so we feel a desire to go back to school, to get back to our roots; the fire can move us upwards, the summer energy can scatter us and spread us quite thin like a love affair that never ends and at a certain point one feels a need for something concrete, to return to habits, to go back home.

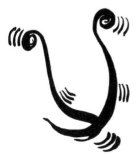

The positions on the floor take us by the hand and guide us through the transitions between summer and autumn. They bring a sense of calm, and ways to enter a season with such different characteristics. They encourage a calm, practical shift.

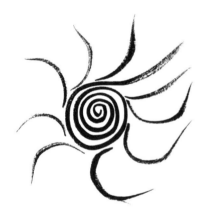

spring summer autumn winter

in spring, hundreds of flowers.
in autumn, the harvest moon.
in summer, a fresh breeze.
snow accompanies you in winter
if you don't have your head stuffed with useless things,
every season is a good season for you

MUMON

translator's note

Yoga is a way of linking up and making connections. Between high and low, front and back, left and right. Between the body and our intentions. Between the sense of freedom and joy, and the sense of security and responsibility. Between where we are and where we might want to be. Joining the actual with the essentially divine. That is the meaning of the word: yoking the present moment with an essential moment, finding union. Linking and making connections through attending to the body and its changing sense of weight and lightness, balance and movement with an attitude of listening and learning. Modestly learning from what we sense through the body. Through the body and with the heart, the feet and the head, and the long spine at the core that runs the length of the body.

We may have some sense of what yoga means, and have been studying it and experiencing the way it helps balance our energies and clears a space for silence and attention within us. Attention to the breath, and awareness of smoothness, and other qualities of the breath are an important part of the link. Breath releases impurities and brings nourishment and lightness. There are teachers and books that help get more fully into the practice of yoga. There are classes, and mats and belts. There is discipline and time, and there is a rhythm which we can eventually sense. We can follow the gift of the breath.

Some do their yoga regularly, and others intend to but somehow fail to find time or space in their lives for this nurture. To offset any tendency we may have (we all have and we tend to do the things we like to do) to immure the practice in habits, and lapse into somewhat mechanical routines. Sandra and Silvia's book guides us into deepening our practice and playing with it through a process of continual acclimatisation. Yoga as inner questioning. This helps avoid getting stuck in our ways, or turning off some qualities of the heart, or some range of impulse or sense of listening. Sandra and Silvia's book has provided an ingenious set of practices in accordance with the tendencies of the seasons — using that special energy. Not going contrary to it, or ignoring it, or brushing it off — but changing pace, tuning in to the particular qualities that time of year brings to the fore, and letting the body become permeable and participate in the changing seasons. They can also be called Spring, Growing, Harvest and Trial — according to the Original I Ching Oracle translated under the auspices of The Eranos Foundation by Rudolf Ritsema and Shantena Augusto Sabbadini.

Whatever the yoga tradition, whatever the pattern of practice, or the novelty of yoga may be, this illustrated book revives a kindled feeling, a fuller sense of being settled into the changes the seasons bring, and enjoying practice with renewed resourcefulness and unexpected qualities of attention.

Ann Colcord

about the authors

Sandra Sabatini started to study yoga in Florence with Dona Holleman in 1975 and was part of her group of yoga teachers for some years which met at Bacchereto where Dona lived and Sandra soon moved. It was a wonderful time of discovery. Some years later she met Vanda Scaravelli and began a journey under her guidance which has not ended. In those years many teachers were seeking a wise and intelligent voice able to instil the fascination of sensing and listening into yoga. Vanda reawakened the intense passion for practice in her pupils that also animated her. In 1986 Sandra was invited to London by Mary Stewart to show her many pupils the approach Vanda had developed in teaching yoga. 'No ambition and infinite time', she often repeated, to keep the practice utterly simple. Later, in retreats offered by Thich Nhat Hanh, Sandra discovered the walking meditation again which Vanda had practiced all along the road to Fiesole, and brought this into her practice. For more than thirty years Sandra has been teaching in Germany, England, Finland, Israel and most recently in India. She lives in Campiglia in Tuscany, a beautiful medieval village near the sea, where she holds residential courses.

Silvia Mori was born and lives in Florence, Italy. Her path with yoga began at Rishikesh, in India, 30 years ago, then she studied with different teachers and found her resonance with Sandra Sabatini and Mary Stewart.
She widened her experience through the practice of Tai Chi Chuan first, and then with Chinese Medicine and its practices. Her studies in Shiatsu started in Italy and put her in touch with body/mind workers from many countries. Throughout her teaching she stresses the importance of auto-massage as a health practice.

She teaches both shiatsu and yoga, also through seminars in places close to Nature offer the chance to practice yoga fully in touch with the Earth and the other Elements. She continues to deepen her studies and practice through the retreats of Thich Nhat Hanh and other meditation traditions. Her research carries forward the integration of movement, breath and awareness.

Monica Smith was born in Italy. She is a musician, teacher and consultant. She collaborates with Carrie Tuke promoting Yoga & Sound, an experiential study and research of breath, gravity and movement. She is an Ohashiatsu graduate and has been studying with American music therapist Awahoshi Kawan and musician and acupuncturist Fabien Maman. She works in London, where she resides, and Italy.

Chloë Fremantle is a painter, illustrator and yoga teacher. She exhibits regularly, and is based in West London. She has illustrated several books, including Sandra Sabatini's *Breath* and her own *Yoga Practice Handbook*. Sandra Sabatini was her first Yoga teacher in 1978 in Florence. From 1982-2002 she worked closely with Mary Stewart in London, who trained her to teach Yoga. She now teaches classes and workshops, and directs the London Yoga Teacher Training Course Group.

Ann Colcord is the London Director of the British American Educational Foundation and the Honorary Secretary of the CG Jung Analytical Psychology Club, London. Her translation from the Italian of Michele Spina's *West of the Moon* won a John Florio prize; and was followed by *Night* and *Sleep: A Utopian Bestiary* by the same author. She is currently writing about cupboards and closets.

notes

1 The exact location of this point is in a valley at the centre of the sole of each foot two thirds from the back of the heel (excluding toes), between the II and III metatharsal joint. It is the 'Sparkling Spring' also indicated on the acupunture meridians maps as Yongquan, or Kidney1.

2 The Qi, or Ki, or Prana, or Pneuma is the Vital Energy that flows inside the body, where matter and energy meet, inside vessels called Meridians or Channels, in every part of the body ... an endless stream that is the source of our being.

3 The ischia are the bony parts of the pelvis that contact the ground or the chair when we are seated and transfer the weight permitting the alignment of the spinal column without any effort (the ileum and the pubis are the other parts of the pelvis).

4 Chinese medicine distinguishes between five phases of energy. This model (called the '5 Elements' or the '5 movements') refers to the cycle of seasons and is articulated in a series of relationships: associations with climate, food, directions, parts of the body, energy channels and internal organs, colours and so forth. In addition to the four seasons and the four directions the Earth is present as a fifth movement and direction 'towards the centre'. In a more ancient tradition the Earth was placed at the centre of a circle representing the cycle of seasons, it later became considered in some traditions as a fifth season, corresponding to 'late summer' and positioned between summer and autumn; in other traditions it was identified as an 18 day phase between the fulcrum of one season and the season following, corresponding to the moments of the solstices and equinoxes. In addition to Metal, which expresses itself with autumnal characteristics there is Water-Winter, Wood-Springtime, Fire-Summer. This model is not only part of Chinese traditional medicine, but part of the whole traditional Chinese way of thinking, from diet to architecture. Many of the names of practices used in this book come from the Chinese tradition and correspond to the names of the 'micro-seasons' as Giulia Boschi presented them in her essay *La radice e i fiori*. For further study, see Diane Connelly's book *Agopuntura tradizionale: La legge dei 5 elementi*.

selected bibliography

Basho's Narrow Road – Spring and Autumn Passages
translated from the Japanese with annotations by Htroski Sato
Stone Bridge Press, Berkeley, Ca 1996

The Complete Poems by Emily Dickinson
Faber & Faber, 1970

The Gateless Gate: The classic book of Zen Koans by Koun Yamada
Wisdom Publications, Boston 2004

Medicina Cinese: La radice e i Fiori by Giulia Boschi
Erga edizioni, 1998

Traditional Acupunture: The Law of the Five Elements
by Dianne M. Connelly, 1975

The Long Road Turns to Joy: A guide to Walking Meditation
by Thich Nhat Hanh
Parallax Press, Berkeley, CA, 1985

Centering
transcribed by Paul Reps
First Turtle edition,1957

Awakening the Spine by Vanda Scaravelli
Harper Collins, 1991

also by **Sandra Sabatini** *from* **Pinter & Martin**

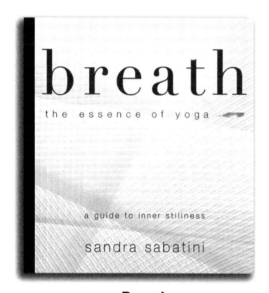

Breath
Paperback | ISBN 978-1-905177-09-7

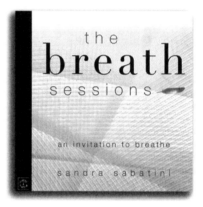

The Breath Sessions
Audio CD | ISBN 978-1-905177-14-1

Sandra Sabatini's *Breath* is full of insights and images, distilled from her yoga classes, to help you learn how to listen to the breath and how to approach some simple positions.

Whether you are a complete beginner or already practice yoga, these subtle, gentle suggestions can guide you naturally to a deeper appreciation of the essence of yoga.